A Journey Through Breast Cancer.

Your Resilient Self

**To the Point
Transformational Handbooks**

Personal Development

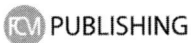 PUBLISHING

Copyright © Jacqueline Mansell 2024
ISBN 978-1-914529-90-0
A CIP catalogue record
for this book is available from the British Library
First printed 2024
Published by FCM PUBLISHING
www.fcmpublishing.co.uk

Also, by Jacqueline Mansell

Resilience A Choice for Everyday Living
Bullying and Harassment of Adults
Influencing and Interpersonal Effectiveness

To the Point – Special Edition

Contents

Appendices

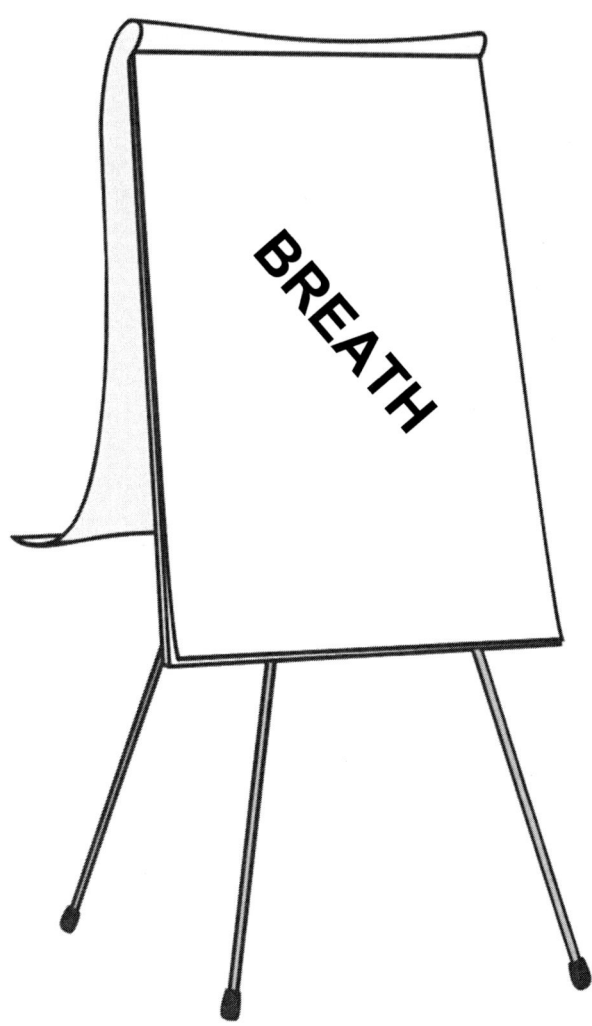

Introduction
A Journey Through Breast Cancer
Thoughts for Coping & Resilience

In the autumn of 2022, I received a diagnosis of Stage 3 Breast Cancer. Life as I knew it, in an instant changed irrevocably. On a practical level, things moved fast, beginning with visits to hospitals, meetings with Doctors and Nurses, blood tests, scans and even dentistry work ahead of Chemotherapy. Given the swift actions of the medical teams involved and the timetable planned for treatment I too found myself swept up in having to quickly prepare for the business of day to day living for the months ahead. However, while all of this was happening and despite the flurry of daytime activity, in those first weeks I lay in bed at night frightened for the future, and as I dared not to close my eyes, the dead of the night seemed somehow to wrap around me, it felt like a velvet curtain, black, and dark.

The journey from those initial dark days began, there were times when I cried and faltered. For example, walking along the corridor of the Chemotherapy Ward for the first time to face treatment. Of course, it is okay to cry, there are times in most people's lives often associated with loss, when all that is wanted is to retreat, curl up in a ball and sob. **The key factor is about getting up and keeping going, and as is the case sometimes in life, this may just be about treading water and coping day to day** until you can actively move forward.

So, while the Chemotherapy Ward was for me a place of anxiety, it was also a place of inspiration, as listening to other people and learning of their own experience created emotional bonds and engendered support and friendship.

With these points in mind this book has been created to share personal experience, tips and hints combined with psychological insights and tools to help readers through challenging times.

A Special Note

For many years I have had the privilege of teaching, facilitating, and writing about resilience (see Appendix 1, Extract from the 2017 book titled, Resilience: A Choice for Everyday Living).
This current book, A Journey Through Breast Cancer, is about your resilient and courageous self. It has been compiled with the experience of breast cancer at its heart where, until you are ready (and as has been said before in other trying

circumstances) life, for the time being might simply be about 'keeping calm and carrying on'. It uses insights from psychology with the intention of being of benefit to the reader. However, as a psychologist I am also minded that the book has been written from my personal perspective, of my lived experience and shares theories and ideas that as a cis gender woman, I have found useful during a challenging journey. This has been an introspective form of psychology where no reviews or other studies have been carried out. With these thoughts in mind, not all content may be representative across all populations. It should be noted that while the book is aimed at creating meaningful and positive impacts, everyone's story will be different. I am also minded that there are different types, grades, and categories of breast cancer plus countless treatment pathways. Everyone travelling the journey will have their own story with different reactions to drugs, surgery etc. However. taking into account these considerations, the aim of this handbook is to:

- Share personal experience.
- Recognise the difference between simply coping and effective coping and resilience skills.
- Enhance personal self-awareness.
- Support positive expectations.
- Aid in reducing anxiety.

- Help with maintaining morale.
- Provide practical tips and ideas.
- Provide an insight for others, such as friends and family.
- Plan goals.

About To the Point Books

'To the Point' are books, which have been developed and written with different readers in mind, but in all cases designed for practical and easy use. These quick to read behavioural skills handbooks typically encapsulate experience and knowledge drawn together throughout a career supporting the development of individuals and organisations. This Special Edition To the Point book shares observations, and personal understanding and experience relating to a journey through breast cancer including psychological theory that was used to get through. For example, identifying areas of control (see Part 2 Locus of Control), maintaining a positive frame of mind (see quotations shared throughout the book), recognising life events where difficult situations had been overcome in the past etc.

To the Point handbooks provide you with straightforward access to theories, ideas and frameworks proven to achieve results, account for behaviour and which can be integrated into the lived experience.

The style of To the Point Books enables different levels of engagement at different points throughout:

- **Quotations** provide nuggets of good advice and information which have been neatly summed up by thinkers of the world.
- **Highlighted Key Words (Flipcharts)** are presented as punctuation points with quintessential meaning.
- **Bullet Points** present a practical and succinct read.
- **Case Studies** are usually to be found in 'To the Point' books. For this particular book, personal experience, insights, and anecdotes are recounted throughout by the author. So, providing a single descriptive case study.
- **Suggested Shopping Lists** have been included in this book. They contain an assortment of miscellaneous items as an aide to help you plan and prepare.

The handbook format and style of layout has great advantages as it eliminates the 'filler'. Meaning that it is useful for people who do not want to spend a lot of time reading, the research has been done and you reach the 'gold seam' of knowledge and ideas immediately.

'To the Point' Books are ideal for:

- Individuals who would like to increase their personal knowledge and understanding.
- Organisations who wish to provide tool books for different people.
- People who want to learn quickly.
- Discovering ideas, information, and concepts to provide a springboard to further exploration.

"Courage must be the harder.
Heart the keener.
Spirits the greater as our strength wanes."

The Beowulf Poet

Part One.

Receiving the bad news

Your Unknown Self (The Johari Window)

The Nadir

"*You must do the thing you think you cannot do.*"

Eleanor Roosevelt

The Johari Window

We begin with a useful tool developed during the 1950's by psychologists Joseph Luft and Harrington Ingham who devised a model for self-discovery which, as will be seen can be applied to the breast cancer journey. This psychological tool is typically used with respect to interpersonal relations as a means to get people talking, to facilitate personal disclosure and elicit feedback. Luft and Ingham identified four different aspects of the self: The Open Self, The Blind Self, The Hidden Self, and the Unknown Self. In order to help conceptualise this idea Luft and Ingham presented the four parts as being like a window divided into four glass panes. These facets of the self may be known **or** unknown to our own selves or to others.

The Open Self

❖ This facet of the person is known to our own selves and known to others. We may display traits such as being trustworthy, calm, and caring, jovial, and fun which are clear to see and open to others.

The Hidden Self

❖ This is an area of the self where a façade is maintained so hiding aspects of one's identity, personality, secrets, fears, emotions, opinions. Matters may be concealed from others such as personal history or mental struggles.

The Blind Self

❖ This aspect of the self is unknown to our own selves but perceived, identified, or observed in us by other people. For example, we may consider ourselves as witty while others see us as obtuse. We might underestimate our abilities while others see us as very capable.

The Unknown Self

❖ In this quadrant we have yet to learn of our potential, of personal gifts such as competence, untapped skills, courage etc. Or yet to recognise our unconscious needs and desires, our motivations, and drivers. Equally, other people do not know what we are capable of.

For all of us there is an Unknown Self, for none of us knows what we will be like 5, 10, 20 years from now. As the Author Thomas Pynchon wrote in reference to the challenges faced by the individuals in his novel, V, 'You wait. Everyone has an

Antarctic'. The question is whether, in the words of Rudyard Kipling we can *'meet with triumph and disaster just the same'*.

And so, on the news of my diagnosis, as I faced my Antarctic, the panes of the Johari Window were about to be opened.

I was able to use the Johari Window to identify strengths: What I knew about myself (the Open Self) was that I have a reasonably sensible approach to things, I'm organised and patient and so these were attributes that I could draw on for the road ahead.

Regarding my Unknown Self, I had no idea how I would cope with the medical procedures that faced me. One of my immediate thoughts (silly as it may sound, and even vain to some) was how would I be without my long hair which, for so many years had for me, been a big part of my identity? Of course, my greatest question of concern to the medical team was the big one about what the future held…

In terms of the Hidden Self, some people might want to open that window: With such a diagnosis, disclosing information, thoughts, feelings, experiences that have been withheld or suppressed may be important. For some, sharing aspects of the private self may bring peace or even perhaps, redemption (who hasn't seen the last chance confession in typical Hollywood movies).

I will return to examples of the Johari Window later on in the book. In the meantime, you may wish to use the Johari Window as a tool for self-reflection and think about your different selves.

Exercise Exploring the Open Self

Appendix 2 provides a list with examples of Johari Window adjectives used to help people to think about aspects of themselves, simply tick those qualities that apply to you, and you may find that heightened self-awareness will create within you a degree of positivity, identify areas where you may need some support and help towards getting you through. You may also wish to remind yourself and list the times when you have successfully overcome difficulties, when you have achieved results and when you have put a brave foot forward. With this knowledge you can add to your confidence and leverage your strengths

It's going to be tough, but you can do this!

The Nadir (the low point)

The Psychologist Abraham Maslow describes a Peak Experience as one of highest fulfilment and happiness. The opposite is a Nadir Experience which is about coming up against a low point, suffering an experience which is traumatic, distressing, unpleasant, harrowing.

The Nadir Experience is the worst experience or worst time of your life. The news of breast cancer may be such an experience and is likely to invoke a range of feelings:

- ◆ Your response to the diagnosis might be:
  - ❖ You can't think straight.
  - ❖ Confusion.
  - ❖ Panic.
  - ❖ Anxiety.
  - ❖ Catastrophizing (focussing on a succession of worst-case scenarios).
  - ❖ Anger.
  - ❖ A sense of loss.
  - ❖ Denial.
  - ❖ Fear.
  - ❖ Dread.
  - ❖ Loneliness.
  - ❖ Depression.

- The complexity of the mind means that emotions can come into play even before we are consciously aware of what is happening (the Limbic System). In turn this can develop into automatic behaviours and so on diagnosis the spontaneous physical expression of emotions might be:

  - ❖ Not listening.

  - ❖ Withdrawal.

  - ❖ A sense of being totally overwhelmed.

  - ❖ Shaking.

  - ❖ Dizziness.

  - ❖ Nausea.

  - ❖ Crying.

  - ❖ Words of anger.

- When being diagnosed:

  - ❖ Try to listen.

❖ Try to understand what is being said by asking for more details.

❖ Be considerate to the individuals or team who are giving you the news. For while they are professionals who are trained to give bad news, they are human too (in other words, *don't shoot the messenger*).

◆ Our mental health and physical health are interrelated, and it is worth noting that the force of our emotions can be so great that they upset other drives such as:

❖ Hunger.

❖ Levels of hydration / being dehydrated.

❖ Sleep.

❖ The will to live.

For myself, the initial biopsy results coincided with catching a really bad cold, the worst I'd had in years. My mental and physical health had orchestrated to bring me even further down!

If your emotions take over your normal good sense, 'don't beat yourself up'. Now the challenge is to tap into your <u>logical, concentrated, rational thoughts,</u> find within yourself the capacity to deal with the situation, adapt, be flexible and **get organised for the months ahead.**

Part Two.

Pressure and Stress

Personal Forcefield Analysis

Locus of Control

"*Organize and execute around priorities.*"

Stephen Covey

The daily business of life does not stop with your diagnosis. While you are occupied with visiting the hospital for various scans, blood tests and meeting with different medical teams, there are still bills to be paid, household chores to be undertaken, tasks to be maintained such as annual insurance renewals, the car MOT etc. Indeed, my own diagnosis coincided with the gas boiler breaking down and the frustration of trying to challenge an estimated gas statement arising from the big hike in energy prices that took place in 2022. However, these events led to a useful piece of learning: The call to the energy company meant the usual frustrating customer experience of telephone menu options, being put on hold, repeating information to customer services etc. By the time I got off the phone I was thoroughly fed up! I was reminded:

You can't get stressed about everything.

Choose and list the things that you are going to get stressed about.

So, what is stress? **Stress at a causal level** is the pressure, the forces placed upon us, or we perceive to be upon us. Stresses can weigh upon us for a short or long period of time. Think of it like this, a balloon or a tyre being pumped full of air, the right amount of pressure and everything is okay, too little air and the tyre or balloon is empty and deflates but filled up with too much air the tyre or balloon explodes. Pressures can come from sources that are psychological (mental/emotional), social or physical.

The cause, namely stressors. **can produce an effect,** which in turn manifests as psychological stress and tension. (See: Resilience. A Choice for Everyday Living Pages 29-41 for other information).

Personal Force Field Analysis

The Psychologist Kurt Lewin recognised that different forces create tension upon us and so developed a model for exploring those factors called Force Field Analysis. This framework is sometimes depicted as being like a Playground Seesaw with one side bringing things down the other side raising things up (Hindering/Helping or Driving Change/Resisting Change).

- **Forces/factors that may cause/increase personal tension/stress during the journey through breast cancer:**
    - ❖ Fear of the medication, of Chemotherapy, Radiotherapy surgery etc.
    - ❖ Assumptions that you will get side effects from the treatment.
    - ❖ Other people's reaction to your news.

❖ Your own reaction to other people's behaviour.

❖ Interpersonal relations with health professionals (their approach and manner may not chime with yours).

❖ Late or re-arranged GP, hospital appointments.

❖ Visiting the hospital in terms of an unfamiliar layout, limited car-parking, access to public transport hubs, the location of wards etc.

❖ Transport to the hospital (managing how you are going to get there and back).

♦ **Forces/factors that may mitigate/decrease personal tension/stress during the journey through breast cancer:**

❖ As mentioned earlier, choosing

those things that you are going to get stressed about.

❖ Mental control and mental outlook. For example, positive self-talk. Looking forward to the end of treatment e.g., planning an event or trip away. (I kept counting down the weeks with the goal of a simple visit to a local restaurant).

❖ Finding out about your treatments. Researching and reading about the illness (I found that literature provided during consultations was very informative).

❖ Taking the opportunity (if available) to engage with or use facilities provided by the staff of Macmillan Cancer Support and other cancer specialist organisations.

❖ Reducing contact with the people that cause you stress.

❖ Maintaining contact with the people that you like.

❖ Doing a 'recce' of the hospital, checking out transport arrangements, obtaining maps, guides, and timetables.

❖ Having provisions ready for the weeks/months ahead (particularly when your immune system is low, and you can't get out).

❖ Preparing a shopping list of different things to buy which may be out of the ordinary such as a wig etc.

❖ Finding things that will occupy your mind that don't require a lot of physicality such as books that you have long wanted to read, puzzles, magazine subscriptions, Netflix, and other subscription services, downloads, Podcasts. perhaps some box sets, DVDs etc.

❖ Doing gentle exercise.

❖ Electing to let things go a little such as cutting down on housework, reducing laundry by wearing clothes a little longer etc.

❖ Getting rest.

You may wish to examine the positive and negative forces which impact upon your present state and will help you to achieve your desired state (in my case I just wanted to focus everything towards recovery).

An Exercise for Personal Forcefield Analysis

As a quick and simple approach to Force field Analysis, first make a list of all the things that could hold you back or are likely to be unfavourable to your current situation then second, list all of the things that will drive you towards your desired state. Within both lists you might want to give each of the factors that you have identified a score in terms of importance e.g. 1 being least important while 10 is very important. These scores will enable you to prioritise and provide a springboard for setting goals, plans, and action. As your journey continues and as the path may veer with different treatments or other challenges, you might wish to revisit and reposition the forces towards changing circumstances. For myself, in the early days being organised was a feature of my list to drive me towards my desired state. However, as my strength has begun to return, the ability to say no and to avoid bad energies has become important.

Locus of Control

The American Psychologist Julien Rotter developed a theory with respect to an individual's belief or perception over the level of control they exercise over personal life events. This model was described as a Locus of Control and presented as a continuum whereby there is a high sense of Internal Control at one end of the spectrum and a recognition of a high level of External Control at the other end of the scale.

People with a tendency towards a high level of internal control believe that they can personally play a considerable part in outcomes and that they have greater agency to influence events. At the other end of the spectrum, people with a high sense of external control see life as external forces over which they have little control.

When you receive a cancer diagnosis it is perhaps only human to feel that you have little control. Of course, there are some things that are suddenly out of your control but there are things over which you do have control:

- Locus of Control. Areas where you may have little or limited control:
  - How the disease will develop within you.
  - Test results.
  - Your initial physical reaction to chemicals, drugs, and other treatments.
  - Other people's reaction and behaviour to the news of your diagnosis.
  - Mood swings which simply come

over you ('Sometimes you eat the bear and sometimes the bear eats you!").

- ◆ Locus of Control. Areas where you have some control:

  - ❖ Accepting your mood swings and emotions. You are likely to be very fatigued and feel ill. Sometimes you are going to be in a state of despair become angry, sad or cry. You are human – it's okay – understand that these states of being will pass. Additionally, if things get tough you can reach out to the medical team or other specialist cancer agencies.

  - ❖ Recognising that you are in good hands. You have the support and care of highly trained medical specialists, including oncologists and surgeons.

❖ Reading and researching the illness. Particularly taking note of pamphlets/booklets issued during consultations or available through Macmillan Cancer Support.

❖ Taking medication and following advice and treatment as prescribed by your consultant etc.

❖ Being honest with the medical team regarding any lifestyle questions. For example, how much you drink or smoke.

❖ Self-health checks. For example, monitoring your daily temperature, as advised. Noting changes to your physical self and alerting your medical support team.

- ❖ Diet, eating and keeping yourself hydrated.

- ❖ Lifestyle, how to some extent, you occupy your time.

- ❖ Who you decide to tell about your condition outside of the medical staff.

- ❖ How you are going to approach hospital visits and your impact on others.

- ❖ Getting organised ahead of treatment. For example, having in place matters related to finance, monies for travelling to and from hospital etc. Arrangements for shopping. Arrangements for work.

- ❖ Our attitude towards the illness, surrender or fight.

An exercise to identify your own Locus of Control.

At the top of a page draw a horizontal line, on the left side of the line write the number 0, this end of the line denotes where you have no control over things (External Locus of Control). At the other end of the line write the number 10, this end of the line denotes where you have total control over things (Internal Locus of Control). In between the numbers 0 and 10 and equally spaced, write the numbers 1 – 9.

Next, using the numbers as you points of reference and underneath the line, list vertically those things over which you have no control through to those things over which you have total control.

In my own case, for example, towards one end of the spectrum I could take control of my thoughts and so I got hold of a little white board and wrote a list of positive thoughts which I hung on the wall.

Plan and Prepare

Special Shopping List No1.

Special Shopping List No1

A Notepad and Pen

When having consultations or treatment you may want to keep notes as it is so easy to forget things when there is such a lot to take in (and if you should suffer 'Chemo Brain Fog' and your capacity to think is not as sharp as usual). Plus, you may wish to keep a note of questions as they arise throughout your day (or night) in order that you can ask your consultant for info.

A4 Diary (Preferably including a Year Planner)

Use your diary and planner to plot out your treatment pathway and in this way, you can see a tentative end goal date and tick off milestones in between. As you become in tune with your body your diary will also be useful for recording changes or special notes.

A Ring Binder and a Box File

A ring binder is a handy place to keep hospital appointment cards and letters. A box file is useful for storing the different size books, booklets and pamphlets issued during treatment.

An 'Address Book'

Your care may be split between several specialized medical teams, and over the course of your treatment you are likely to be given a lot of different contact details. You may find it useful to organise contacts on your mobile phone into groups, create a database of useful info or jot details into an address book.

N.B. Typically, stationery available at WHSmith or large supermarkets.

Part Three.

(Chemotherapy: Losing your hair, your mind and confidence).

Maintaining a positive mindset

Confidence

"Everyone has a plan until they get punched in the face."

Mike Tyson

The literature provided by my medical team states that: *Chemotherapy for cancer means that anti-cancer drugs are given by injection… or in tablet form to kill or control cancer cells.* There *are more than 80 different anti-cancer drugs.* With this in mind I must reiterate that different people may/will have different experiences of chemotherapy to that which is described here. However, on talking to other patients it would seem chemotherapy is something whereby:

You just have to grind it out.

If you have a forward diary, you can plot out the proposed program of treatment and however many rounds of chemotherapy are planned you can countdown the weeks, giving you hope and knowledge that as far as anticipated:

This is a temporary situation.

As to my own chemotherapy, it was intravenous chemotherapy given via a canular into the hand or arm every three weeks. Treatment took place on an Outpatients Ward and lasted several hours. Each treatment was preceded by a hospital visit a few days earlier to provide blood which was checked to see if chemotherapy could go ahead as planned. At each round of chemotherapy, I was also supplied with a cocktail of medication, including steroids etc with many to counteract or diminish chemotherapy side-effects such as anti-sickness, anti-nausea, heartburn tablets etc plus injections to be self-administered to the stomach each night for seven days per round of chemotherapy.

It didn't take long for noticeable side effects to kick in from being sick, to constant waves of nausea, feeling extremely tired and fatigued, heartburn, inflamed sore mouth etc and of course within weeks the dreaded hair loss occurred. Taste buds changed, there was a heightened sense of smell and food normally enjoyed was no longer wanted one month but wanted the next! There is no advise I can give on recommended foods, as for myself and the other patients that I met, food and drink was just so difficult to get right. As the months went on, I was advised that I would feel that I had been 'flattened' and wow, that advice was so right! Pain to fingers and toenails occurred as they softened and peeled away while aches to the bones and muscles set in.

While chemotherapy produced physical side effects, something discussed when visiting the ward was a shared experience in terms of brain fog, self-doubt, and a sense of depression.

Maintaining a positive mindset.

Focussing on a Life Well Lived

Chemotherapy came with a lot of rest time and

with sleeplessness. It is in these hours when doubt, regret (for things you have and haven't done) and sadness can invade thoughts. Therefore, **try to keep a positive mindset.** One of the ways in which you can do this is by maintaining your self-esteem (or raising it while feeling low). This means recognising your worth through positive evaluation. Here we **focus on a life well lived.**

- In broad terms, the Psychologist Shigehiro Oishi (and plus others) has identified that a life well lived can be divided into three categories:
  - ❖ A happy, hedonic life.
  - ❖ A meaningful life (Eudaimonia).
  - ❖ A psychologically rich life.

- A happy, hedonic life. Think of the things that have given you general life satisfaction or an inner sense of wellbeing or peace:

- ❖ Having positive relationships.

- ❖ Attachments that you have had (for example may be a special person, a loved pet etc).

- ❖ Hobbies and pastimes such as cooking, gardening, crafts, sports, music, reading, arts (for art's sake).

- ❖ Maintaining order in your life. For example, managing your finances, having a stable home and social life.

- ❖ Maintaining life's rituals and treats. For example, regular trips to the hairdressers/beauticians. Lunch or trips out to the pub with friends.

- ❖ Having experiences simply for the sake of enjoyment.

- ❖ A life where you have felt comfort and a sense of security.

- A life that has had meaning and realised potential (Eudaimonia) For example reflect on things such as:

  - The achievements of which you are proud.

  - Your beliefs.

  - Your moral principles.

  - Contributions that you may have made to society. For example, within the different communities that you have occupied, within your family, in your neighbourhood, through your work etc.

  - Your relationships.

  - The skills that you have learned.

  - The experiences that have given you purpose.

  - Contributions that you have made

to the world at large simply through your character and individuality. For example, a positive persona, a kindly word or smile to strangers, lending an ear, being amiable, just by being you!

◆ A psychologically rich life. These may be experiences to think about such as:

❖ The difficulties in life that you have overcome.

❖ How you have dealt with the unexpected.

❖ The different opportunities that you have taken.

❖ The experiences in life that have enabled you to grow and change your perspective. Some may be first hand, lived experience while a change of perspective might have also arisen through vicarious experience. For example, through the achievements of someone else or simply by reading an influential book, watching a movie, reflecting on the arts etc.

❖ All of the experiences that have given you a sense of being engaged, excited, of being alive.

Maintaining a positive mindset.

Confidence and Self-Concept

One of the expressions used by people when chatting on the chemotherapy ward was 'chemo-brain'. It seemed a shared experience that we had were with problems with cognition and things like memory recall. Indeed, I felt like a three-year-old when I was talking to my surgeon and kept repeating myself while I was barely able to string together a sentence! This phenomenon, like losing your hair can be a knock to self-concept and confidence. Your self-concept is your complete personal reference point in terms of who you are, and this can be weakened when confidence is lowered i.e., belief in your own abilities, your ability to solve problems, your sensitivity to the cues and signals presented by the world around you, your capability in terms of making choices and making decisions. When confidence is weakened personal power can feel as if lowered, you feel as though you cannot do things and you may not even want to try.

<u>Some Exercises to strengthen your confidence and self-concept:</u>

- ◆ Exercise One:

    - ❖ Write one or more positive words that you would use to describe yourself.

    - ❖ Write one or more positive word that others would use to describe you.

- ◆ Exercise Two:

    - ❖ Focus on a life well lived. Make a list related to A happy life, a meaningful life, and a psychologically rich life.

    - ❖ Make a list of your skills.

    - ❖ Make a list of your achievements.

    - ❖ Make a list of your personal strengths.

♦ Exercise Three:

Complete the following statements:

  ❖ Wanted for always being…

  ❖ Wanted for living by the slogan…

  ❖ The positive advantage of being me is…

Other ways to strengthen your confidence and self-concept:

♦ Self-awareness: Reflect on those times when you have 1. Felt lacking in confidence and the times that you have 2. Felt confident. What was the difference that made the difference?

Think of the times when your confidence was high and use this knowledge to give you a firm footing as you take steps forward.

- Self-talk: Give yourself some encouraging messages. For example:
  - ❖ You are as bright and capable as most people.
  - ❖ **YOU CAN DO THIS.**
- Engage in relaxation exercises which will help to relax and calm the mind.
- Finally, remind yourself that you won't always feel or look tired, your hair will grow back, and brain-fog will dissipate.

In the words of Winston Churchill:

"When we face with a steady eye the difficulties which lie before us, we may derive confidence from remembering those we have already overcome".

Plan and Prepare

Special Shopping List No2.

Preparing for Chemotherapy

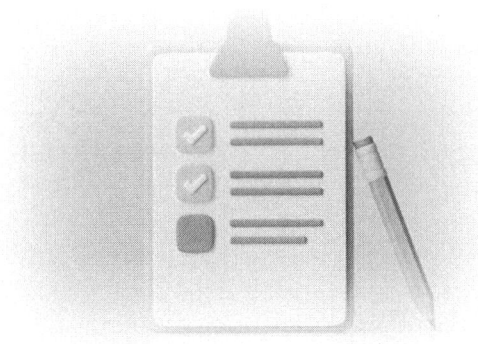

Special Shopping List No2

Baby Shampoo

When you lose your hair, your head will feel different and may be irritated. (I felt uncomfortable about touching my bald head and so I also purchased **a sponge** in order to apply shampoo etc.) *(Baby Shampoo and Sponge available from Boots)*

A Wig

Before buying a wig, you may wish to check if there are any special NHS schemes or suppliers to help towards purchasing a wig. (*For myself, information was available at the hospital that I was attending).*

Head Coverings

The type of head covering is likely to depend on the time of year. My chemotherapy spanned the winter months, and my hair didn't start growing until well into the summer months but my advice here is that while you have no or little hair, have a lining of silky/satiny fabrics directly against your skin as your head may be feeling irritable *(I found a good selection of mob caps etc on Amazon particularly a brand called FocusCare Sleep Cap (Sold by Beauty Turban) which, I found suitable for daytime wear (although advertised for night wear)).* Plus, your head (likely being exposed for the first time since you were born may feel the cold) and so at home I found Turbie Twist Towels really useful and easy to wash.

Eyebrow Stencil Pack

It may be an odd thing when you see yourself without eyelashes and eyebrows for the first time. Therefore, while it might seem trivial an Eyebrow Stencil pack is useful in order to apply reasonably looking false eyebrows. (Chatting on the chemotherapy ward, changes to appearance were very important to patients). (*The Eyebrow pack I used was the W7 Brow Bar Eyebrow Set (www.w7makeup,co,uk)*)

A Bucket

The unfortunate reality is that chemotherapy can make you feel sick and make you actually sick.

Boxes of Tissues and Paper Towels

Face and Body Wet Wipes

In the first days after chemotherapy has been administered you may be feeling extremely fatigued and may not feel like bathing or showering.

Drinks such as water, sparkling water, Lucozade, Tonic Water etc

Your mouth feel may be different to usual or can be very sore. (If you like hot drinks such as tea and coffee you may find they are not as enjoyable as usual).

Drinking Straws

The initial rounds of chemotherapy left me feeling weak and for the first day or so afterwards I struggled to lift my head to drink. Drinking straws bought at the local supermarket proved really helpful for keeping up fluids and taking small sips of drink.

Mouthwatering sweets like fruit flavoured Tic-tac's, fruit jellies etc

While I don't want to encourage tooth decay and dietary advice can be sought from your medical team, I did notice when chatting with other patients that sweets were a bit of a comfort in terms of the horrible mouth feel left by chemotherapy. Some people wanted sour sweets while another said that she craved lemon flavours. I found myself frantically searching for the 'red ones' in bags of jellies :-)

A Clear Cosmetic/Wash Bag

You may have a lot of different packets of pills. I found it useful to be able store packets of pills in a rigid clear bag *(I used a clear travel bag that I had previously bought for going on holiday from M&S)* as it was then organised, and medication was easy to find. (I had a great many pills to take throughout the day. You may find it useful to write out a list or spreadsheet which can be ticked off throughout different times of the day).

Part Four.

Your personal impact

Friendships revealed.

"Let us be grateful to people who make us happy; they are the charming gardeners who make our souls blossom."

Marcel Proust

Your Personal Impact

Many years ago, while teacher training, I wrote about random strangers temporarily forming groups and came across a neat description:

'A group is a collection of individuals ploughing their own and different furrows, whilst a team is a collection of individuals jointly ploughing the same furrow(s).'

Unknown

Being part of a group of people can engender a sense of belonging, common membership and even attachment. It is well documented that being part of (an 'in') group can play a role in individual wellbeing and achievement.

When you are visiting the hospital, you will inevitably engage in interpersonal relations and likely to be in temporary group situations, be it in a waiting room or on a ward. You will be with people from different walks of life, across different generations, differently abled, race, gender, etc, people with different types of cancer etc. Some people seeking cancer prevention (for example, I met a woman during surgery who had undertaken a preventative mastectomy for a genetic condition), some people for curative and some people for palliative care. Some people will be anxious, others fearful and many people I spoke to were very, very tired as nighttime sleep quality had been completely disrupted.

For myself, initially I was frightened and didn't want to identify with the environment. This wasn't where I saw myself, cancer happened to other people, for after all I was a long-time distance runner who only weeks before diagnosis had completed a newly organised running event. However, I quickly learned that it was an extraordinary space with very special people, both in terms of medical teams and patients.

How you can positively impact the environment.

Recognise that your emotional state will not only have a personal effect but also an effect upon others. Therefore:

- Plan to try to arrive in plenty of time for appointments. This will mean that you have time to find where you're going and decompress from your journey.

- Practice patience (as I say in the first book on resilience, supermarkets have queues, when you are in a hurry and driving, you will inevitably meet with roadworks etc). Appointments can run late for a variety of reasons. You may wish to clear the decks either side of appointment times as this will relieve you of demands and pressure. You can than put your focus into your appointment and relax a little. For example, I found out on one occasion the person having the doctor's appointment before me had been given the very worst news. On the day of one of my surgeries it turned out that delays and rearrangements to surgery times had been needed due to a situation that had been necessary for the medical team to manage earlier that day.

❖ When attending consultations perhaps take with you a Thermos Travel Mug with a hot drink or carry a soft drink for while you are waiting. You might also want to take a little snack (e.g., a bar of chocolate, don't be anti-social and take a cheese and onion sandwich ha ha!).

❖ When attending long stints of chemotherapy (or other treatments such as I had with additional infusions) you might find it useful to have music to listen to or a book, Kindle, or magazine to read. One of the women on the surgical ward had her iPad with her and played games and watched films.

♦ Be sensitive to the mood in the room.

♦ Be self-aware while also being observant of others.

   ❖ Think about the type of energy you are giving out to other people with your body language if for example, you don't even bother to look up from your phone or book etc.

   ❖ Communicate with other people, this might simply be with a smile or by opening a conversation with innocuous questions such as how the journey to hospital was or comments about the weather. Be self-aware in terms of listening and observant of 'turn-taking' during conversation.

If you do get into chatting with other people, it can provide a connection and you may find that bonds are quickly formed which give a safe space to share experiences and concerns or even a bit of light-hearted humour. (It was out of a few short simple conversations that I have met some lovely people who have given encouragement and also been helpful in sharing experiences).

❖ Be prepared to break the awkward silence (those occasions where everyone is feeling self-conscious).

However, show respect, be observant of the fact that some people may not want to talk. Be self-aware and know when to stop talking: Following one of my surgeries, the constant talking by the men in the adjacent ward was a little bonding moment for myself and the women who were sharing the same surgical bay: Not only did it give us some common ground but one of the men in particular had a very loud voice and was quite opinionated so gave us an additional source of fun! He was quite indignant when one of the nurses (in the wee small hours of the morning) finally asked him to get some rest :-)

♦ Be courteous and kind.

  ❖ Being polite and cooperative, saying please and thank you. These little things can smooth the way.

    (A few years ago, a survey was published which listed people not saying thank you in the workplace as a Top 20 complaint, I am sure the same complaint applies outside of the workplace too).

  ❖ Offer appreciation and (genuine) compliments.

One of the features of the chemotherapy ward was a large bell hanging from the wall near to the exit. This bell was rung by patients on completion of all the cycles of their treatment. It proved a terrific way to engender a sense of community and belonging as it was a talking point right from the get-go through to the joy of clapping for people as they rang the bell before leaving.

On the evening that I rang the bell there was a man in the corridor of the waiting area. My emotions left me tearful, and I apologised to the man to which he gave me a hug and replied that he had just started his journey and seeing the bell being rung had given him hope for his own future. Little actions can have a big impact.

<u>Friendships and Relationships Revealed</u>

The news of your diagnosis and months of different treatments may have an effect upon your different relationships, from work associations through to your children (if any), family and intimate partners etc. Earlier, I mentioned the Johari Window, different facets to the self, apply as much to others as to you. Macmillan Cancer Support provide a range of leaflets which give advice and guidance concerning relationships.

However, one of the matters that I want to quickly look at here surrounds a conversation on a ward about friendships.

In some cases, it seemed to be that people such as friends, colleagues, family etc. had distanced themselves from patients or been thoughtless in their actions. Now it may be that you have simply uncovered the truth that someone was all along just a 'fair-weather' friend. On the other hand, the person(s) in question may:

♦ Be in shock and fearful.

♦ Be in denial.

♦ May not know how to cope with what is happening to you.

♦ Lack understanding of what is actually happening.

♦ Know too well what is happening and it has unearthed painful memories.

◆ Want/need to distance themselves from what is happening.

◆ Fear catching the disease.

◆ As strange as you might think, be jealous that you are receiving attention.

◆ Not want the normal comfortable, easy life to be disrupted.

◆ Be concerned that the dynamics of usual roles may be altered. For example, you might always be the one who provides the shoulder to cry on.

◆ Not know what to say.

Dr Sarah Vohra notes that other people and their moods etc. can have a real impact on mental wellbeing. She uses a metaphor relating to the notion of spring cleaning our storage closet of clothes and how we might 'cast a critical eye over our wardrobe'. As you might do a spring clean of your wardrobe you may need to cast careful judgment over other aspects of life and consider why hang on to something. You may choose to take leave and bid adieu.

On the other hand, it can be important to keep friendships and relationships alive. Over the course of a relationship there may have been things that you have valued and been grateful for. Therefore, at a time when you feel ready you may, without fuss or criticism, wish to reach out. A simple message where you suggest a plan such as meeting together for a coffee and cake might just do the trick.

A final note: After initial enthusiasm and offers of help, it can be hard for people to maintain high levels of support and interaction wanes, particularly when they have their own lives going on. However, you may be in for some nice surprises as people outside of your normal circle rally around you.

There are lots of meetings and cancer friendship groups organised through various organisations and it may be that this is a point in life where you find new relationships are forged particularly based upon your shared experience and camaraderie.

"Friendship is a sheltering tree."

Samuel Taylor Coleridge

Plan and Prepare

Special Shopping List No3.

Preparing ahead of surgery

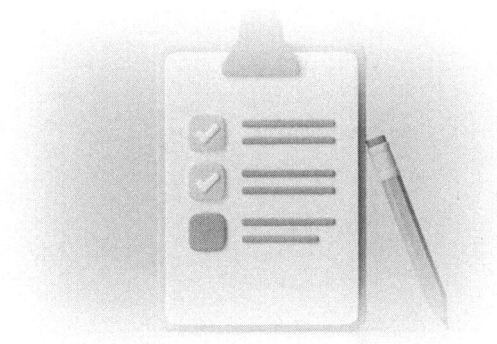

Special Shopping List No3

A Mobile Phone Portable Charger

A Portable Charger will give you confidence that your phone isn't going to run out while you are in hospital.

Button Through Clothing/Tops/Shirts

After surgery you will be in some discomfort and arm movement may initially be limited. Plus, you may have surgical drains attached to your wounds. Therefore, for ease of purpose (particularly when visiting the hospital for post-surgery checks etc.) you may find it easier to wear button through shirts/tops.

Disposable Tableware and Cutlery

When you return home from surgery many household tasks are restricted during the weeks of the recovery period. With limited movement you may find simple tasks like washing-up difficult therefore, to ease your day disposable or compostable tableware *(which I found available at the local supermarket)* can be useful.

Ready Meals

For reasons described above you may wish to plan before surgery by batch cooking and freezing or buying in ready meals or foods that require little preparation. (Alternatively, ready meal delivery services might be something to look into).

Part Five.

The Paradox of Good News

Post Traumatic Growth

"Fear thought is futile worrying over what cannot be averted or will probably never happen."

Winston Churchill

The Paradox of Good News

As chemotherapy drew to a close the next stage in the process began with scans and infusions (as my blood count had not sufficiently recovered), an appointment with the breast clinic to prepare ahead of the operation and a general pre-op appointment. Surgery took place and a few weeks later biopsy results were delivered. The biopsy results showed the spread of cancer into the lymph nodes and so it followed that another operation took place to remove more lymph nodes. Wound checks were carried out throughout, and the management of a surgical drain was not very pleasant.

With so many procedures and the uncertainty of biopsy results, I was given gentle words that (under these circumstances) 'worry serves no purpose'. And so, the day arrived for the second set of lymph node biopsy results.

What a strange day! The news was that while more cancer had been found, as far as possible it had been removed. The medical team had arranged a series of adjuvant therapies to be carried out over forthcoming months and years including radiotherapy, hormone therapy and immunotherapy. To all effects the news that day was good but in the consulting room there was a sense of disbelief and then relief, but the atmosphere was strangely flat...

Emotional Exhaustion - Burnout

Burnout was identified by the Psychologist Christina Maslach and primarily related to the workplace setting. However, it has been widely translated that any emotionally demanding situation where you have to keep going and deal with things otherwise likely to cause distress may leave you feeling exhausted and drained. Burnout can reach a point where a person has simply had enough, they can't take any more, don't care anymore and may even become desensitised and disconnected from their normal self.

The 'Let Down Effect'

The Let Down Effect is when you have been in highly stressful circumstances (think of planning events, dealing with a crisis, being in a job where you are constantly under pressure (in some cases it may be a job you find fulfilling or meeting deadlines that you enjoy) and the situation is over and there is a sort of emptiness, a question of what now? This is the Let Down Effect. It is a phenomenon illustrated with respect to high achieving sports medallists after the rush of training and achieving their goal.

In all circumstances described above stress levels

are likely to have been ramped up to high. Suddenly there is a change and stress hormone levels alter. This phenomenon can quickly take place and in the following period can leave a person susceptible to things like migraine (you may have heard of the 'Weekend Headache' or the 'Holiday Headache'), colds, mood swings or for some people, anxiety (where they are worried that things will happen again), or depression. In most cases symptoms will pass quickly. You may become burnt out or experience the let down effect. For myself, I found I was in my dressing gown for two days after the consultation feeling like I was aching all over and generally unwell.

Recovering your equilibrium

♦ Recognise that this will pass, for the time being the body just hasn't had time to recover from the effects of stress. You have been in a high stress situation.

♦ Talk to other people in order to help you to rationalise your train of thought and put everything into context.

♦ Accept that anxiety may be heightened. (You can still approach the medical team and allay fears).

♦ Do things to relax yourself. This may be specific relaxation techniques, getting absorbed into a hobby, going for a walk or little pleasures and indulgences.

♦ If symptoms such as anxiety do persist or resurface you may need to seek help from your GP.

♦ Be considerate to anyone who has been caring for you as they too may be feeling the same way.

♦ Finally, in the words of those around me:

   'Go out there and enjoy life!'

Post Traumatic Growth

In my 2017 book, Bullying and Harassment of Adults, I talk about post traumatic growth. Post traumatic growth is a psychological response to challenging, traumatic events/situations. There can be situations where individuals disassociate from their trauma or struggle to make sense of what has happened asking why me? On the other hand, post traumatic growth can bring positive change for both individuals and groups.

Post traumatic growth is something that you may experience on your journey through breast cancer. Enlightenment and inspiration may come to you in a flash. Alternatively, years down the line your experience may have a profound effect and move you to change.

Psychologist Steve Taylor talks of transformation through trauma but also describes intense 'awakening experiences' where we might colloquially say that someone has 'seen the light'. Steve Taylor acknowledges that for some people transformation can mean that existing relationships and ways of living break down or change as new identities emerge.

In the context of the breast cancer journey and post traumatic growth, I return again to discuss the panes of the Johari Window. You may find that upon your journey you realise a new reality (for some people this may be a survivor identity), in turn, you develop a new self-awareness. For example, opening up the Unknown Self and discovery strengths you didn't know you had. For myself, I discovered that I could overcome the challenges of procedures such as needles, cannulas, and surgery. As I write this, I am discovering that I am learning to accept my changed body; I am sad for the old one, but I can now look forward to embracing the new. I have had a glimpse of my own mortality and <u>really</u> have learned that life is short and to find happiness in each day.

Equally, in those times where you find yourself reflecting upon your life, you may find that you see things to which you have previously been blind. Elizabeth Grant the Author of Eat, Pray, Love describes how she has 'never seen any life transformation that didn't begin with the person in question finally getting sick of their own bullshit' and maybe that means the BS/nonsense of other people too!

 The Open Self may be strengthened and give you a renewed sense of confidence.

Typically, post traumatic growth is associated with changes such as:

- A new perspective on life.
- A renewed appreciation for life.
- A sense of reinvigoration.
- Greater appreciation for the simple things of life and for each new day.
- An increase in empathy for others.
- An increase in compassion for others.
- Increased appreciation for particular people.
- Greater acceptance of personal vulnerability.
- Increased levels of wisdom.

For some people post traumatic growth can herald a new beginning or provide a platform from which to move forward:

- Making decisions about what is important

in life.

- Reevaluating existing attachments, be they material, emotional, or social.
- Altering assumptions about the world.
- Changing existing behaviours and habits.
- Developing a new attitude.
- Developing new personal boundaries.
- Reevaluating personal identity.
- Becoming the person, they want to be.
- Making career changes.
- Relocating
- Creating a new way of living.
- A prompt to start ticking off the 'Bucket List'.
- Even looking to make dreams come true!

We live and learn.

Part Six.

Survivor Identity

Setting New Goals

"Don't hide your scars. They make you who you are."

Frank Sinatra

Survivor Identity

When I was young, previous generations talked about cancer in a hush hush manner, spoken of furtively with people talking behind their hand. Now the taboo has been lifted and there is a visible level of support for breast cancer: The Pink Ribbon which has become an emblem for breast cancer awareness was co-created by Estee Lauder Cosmetics in the early 1990s. There now exists an annual Breast Cancer Awareness Month, an annual National Cancer Survivor Day and many calls to action, charity walking and running events and other special occasions.

A journey through breast cancer is about more than the illness per se, it may also be about survival (while feeling fatigued and fragile) in terms of things like managing finances, maintaining a job role, navigating relationships with your circle of friends, colleagues, family and loved ones, and of course, coming to terms with changes to the body and body image. Underlying all this may be a fear of cancer reoccurring.

Survivor identity may serve as a way of coping through difficult times. Chats along the way with other patients can provide reassurance in shared experience. Relationships forged with other patients may provide a release through 'gallows' humour. Beyond this, some people may find that as someone whose has first-hand of surviving breast cancer they are able to promote preventative strategies by encouraging friends, family, workmates etc. to be vigilant about changes to their bodies or to attend regular mammograms. Other people might actively get involved in campaigns or wear breast cancer related apparel and items such as the Pink Ribbon.

On the other hand, you may be someone who wants to be private or simply doesn't want to talk about your own lived experience or feelings about your breast cancer for reasons known to you. The time may simply not be right for you, or you might just be the type of person who likes to take a low-key approach. For myself, I didn't want to put my initial diagnosis onto social media, nor did I want to be seen out as I felt very self-conscious about my whole persona.

Each day that passes is a day that you have survived. You may wish to plan a goal for an anniversary date (be it when you were first diagnosed or when you completed treatments) as a marker of how far you have come...

Setting New Goals

As at the date of writing the body of this book I am mindful that my journey continues, I still have radiotherapy to come, energy levels have been lowered and other therapies with their own side effects such as nausea, severe diarrhoea, fever type symptoms and fatigue need to be managed. However, with life slowly returning to a new normal (life now includes daily medication, diarising and attending regular reviews, checkups, the side effects of Lymphedema, and additional treatment, living with the niggle of recurrence and of course a changed body) for me, this is a good point at which to set some future goals.

Goals can be categorised as:

- ♦ Short Term
- ♦ Medium Term
- ♦ Long Term

The span of time between the short, medium, and long term will be different for everyone. For me, an example of goals are as follows:

- ♦ Short Term Goal
  - ❖ *Enjoy some trips out and meet up with friends.*
- ♦ Medium Term Goal
  - ❖ *Restore fitness to previous levels.*
- ♦ Long Term Goal
  - ❖ *Go on a holiday abroad – somewhere warm.*

In keeping with the analogy of a journey, goals provide a directional plan/map of where you are going for which you might want to set objectives. Objectives are typically framed and set using the mnemonic, S.M.A.R.T:

- ♦ **S**pecific
  - ❖ *For example, specifically where do I intend to go on holiday?*

- <u>M</u>easurable

    - ❖ *For example, how much do I intend to spend on a holiday abroad?*

- <u>A</u>chievable

    - ❖ *For example, how much money do I need to go on holiday?*

- <u>R</u>ealistic or <u>R</u>elevant

    - ❖ *For example, why is this goal important? Why is it important for me to go on a holiday abroad?*

- <u>T</u>imebound

    - ❖ *For example, what is the actual date by which I want to go on holiday?*

Next, create an Action Plan and then a To Do List and you will really be on the way to reaching your goals.

An Action Plan is typically set around some key points. As relevant, list your answers to the following:

- What is the action I am going to take?

- How will I complete the action?

- Whose help will I need?

- What additional resources will I need?

- The date I intend to start.

- The date I intend to complete the action.

Finally, you, as someone whose life has been turned upside down will know more than most that while you may have set out plans the reality is that they can meet bumps along the way. Therefore, you also know that you may need to put plans to one side or rearrange priorities. As Ernest Shackleton described, look at any changing circumstances as a new mission.

Keep faith, focus where you can on happiness and in the lyrics of John Lennon remember:

"Life is what happens to you when you're busy making other plans".

Note

This book has been written from a personal appreciation of the breast cancer journey. It is intended to enhance self-awareness and provide psychological theories, models, tips, and ideas as an aide to navigating the breast cancer journey. *(Please note, references to purchases shown in shopping lists are to provide examples only and are not endorsements for products or suppliers).*

The NHS and Macmillan Cancer Support supply excellent literature written to guide and inform as you undertake treatments for breast cancer. **This book is not a substitute for material provided by the NHS, Macmillan Cancer Support etc. and your specialist carers.**

It is also noted that for some people breast cancer may be a long ongoing journey, here, for example, I think of the fortitude and strength of Jane Tomlinson CBE. In addition, some people need additional support to recover from traumatic experiences. With this in mind the expertise of medical and other support groups should always be sought as required.

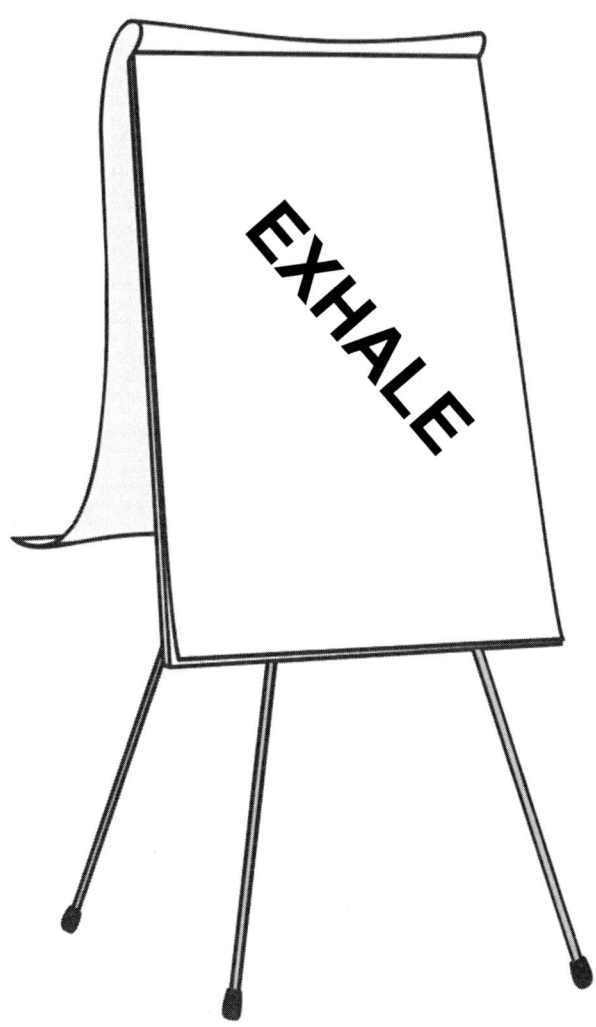

About the Author

Jacqueline Mansell CPsychol., AFBPsS., Chartered FCIPD., FSET., is a Chartered Psychologist who has worked in a career dedicated to learning and development.

During the course of her career Jacqueline has reached many people through her various roles and business and now also brings her accumulated knowledge and expertise to a wider audience through her handbooks.

To the Point handbooks have been designed by Jacqueline to provide a compilation of her reference notes and presentation materials, built over the span of many years. The handbooks cover psychological themes accessible and applicable to everyday living.

Acknowledgements

With a profound thank you for the
National Health Service.

**Special thanks, for his support during this
challenging time, to
Daniel Taylor.**

Thank you to others – you know who you are.

Finding Inspiration in Other People

Finally, along the journey I have found inspiration
in many people. Including, for example, an
interview where the Artist Tracy Emin described
her own battle with cancer. The American
President, John Kennedy who ran a country while
having to take a daily cocktail of prescription drugs
to deal with underlying health conditions.
However, a particularly special note goes out to
Tony Hudgell BEM and to Luke Mortimer (See
project, Band of Builders). Serendipitously, when I
was feeling a bit low, these two young brave
individuals were featured on the TV. Their
courage, spirit and achievements were very
inspirational. I wish them great success as they
move forwards with their lives.

Appendix 1

Extract from Resilience. A Choice for Everyday Living (2017)

Mental control

♦ Being mentally strong.

♦ Mental energy and toughness.

♦ Having personal control.

♦ Inner strength.

♦ Being composed.

♦ Having the strength to do more than just cope.

Mental Outlook

♦ Confidence, self-belief, and efficacy.

♦ An attitude of living life to the full, understanding that change can happen in an instant.

♦ Remaining positive in difficult situations.

♦ Energy (feeling alive, feeling wanted, feeling needed, feeling connected, feeling alert).

♦ Limiting the thinking that brings us down while increasing the thinking that lifts us up.

♦ Being focussed.

♦ Being persistent.

- Being determined to see things through to the end.
- Learning to act, rather than react.

Self-maintenance

- Personal risk management. Strategies and plans to protect yourself for the present and the future.
- Developing knowledge, skills, and capabilities.
- When necessary, having the courage to reach out and ask for help.
- Building and nurturing relationships with other people.

Recovery

- Withstanding stress and pressure.
- Overcoming adverse events and experiences.
- Bouncing back after a difficult/terrible event.
- Recovering easily from hardship.
- Planning and goal setting.

Learning

- Coming through negative situations with more confidence, not less.
- Having a growth mind-set.
- Recovery and survival which results in learning and in turn leads to personal growth.

Appendix 2

The Johari Window Adjectives

- Able
- Accepting
- Adaptable
- Bold
- Brave
- Calm
- Caring
- Cheerful
- Clever
- Complex
- Confident
- Dependable
- Dignified
- Empathetic
- Energetic
- Extroverted
- Friendly
- Giving
- Happy
- Helpful
- Idealistic
- Independent
- Ingenious
- Intelligent
- Introverted
- Kind
- Knowledgeable
- Logical
- Loving

- Mature
- Modest
- Nervous
- Observant
- Organized
- Patient
- Powerful
- Proud
- Quiet
- Reflective
- Relaxed
- Religious
- Responsive
- Searching
- Self-assertive
- Self-conscious
- Sensible
- Sentimental
- Shy
- Silly
- Smart
- Spontaneous
- Sympathetic
- Tense
- Trustworthy
- Warm
- Wise
- Witty

Appendix 3

The Author's Journey through Breast Cancer.
An example of a treatment pathway.

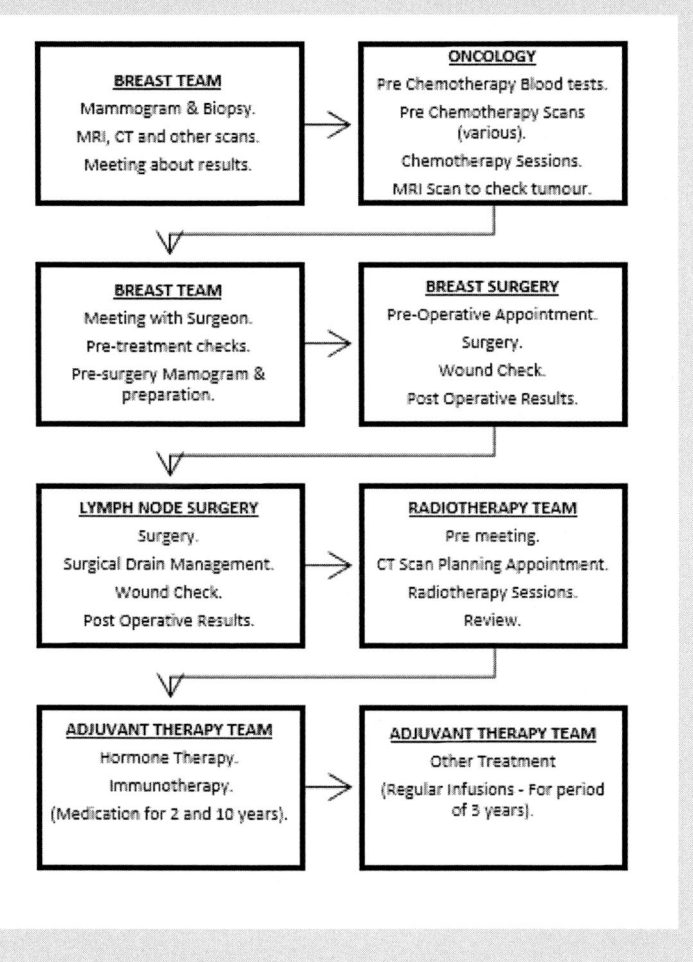